Strain

Grower

Acquired

AF379437

Date

$

| Indica | Hybrid | Sativa |

☐ Flower   ☐ Edible   ☐ Concentrate

Symptoms Relieved

Sweet
Fruity
Floral
Sour
Spicy
Earthy
Herbal
Woodsy

Notes

Effects	Strength
Peaceful	○ ○ ○ ○ ○
Sleepy	○ ○ ○ ○ ○
Pain Relief	○ ○ ○ ○ ○
Hungry	○ ○ ○ ○ ○
Uplifted	○ ○ ○ ○ ○
Creative	○ ○ ○ ○ ○

Ratings ☆ ☆ ☆ ☆ ☆

Strain

Grower

Acquired

Date

$

| Indica | Hybrid | Sativa |

☐ Flower ☐ Edible ☐ Concentrate

Symptoms Relieved

Sweet

Fruity

Floral

Sour

Spicy

Earthy

Herbal

Woodsy

Notes

Effects	Strength
Peaceful	○ ○ ○ ○ ○
Sleepy	○ ○ ○ ○ ○
Pain Relief	○ ○ ○ ○ ○
Hungry	○ ○ ○ ○ ○
Uplifted	○ ○ ○ ○ ○
Creative	○ ○ ○ ○ ○

Ratings ☆ ☆ ☆ ☆ ☆

Strain

Grower

Date

Acquired

$

| Indica | Hybrid | Sativa |

☐ Flower   ☐ Edible   ☐ Concentrate

Symptoms Relieved

Notes

Sweet

Fruity

Floral

Sour

Spicy

Earthy

Herbal

Woodsy

Effects	Strength
Peaceful	○ ○ ○ ○ ○
Sleepy	○ ○ ○ ○ ○
Pain Relief	○ ○ ○ ○ ○
Hungry	○ ○ ○ ○ ○
Uplifted	○ ○ ○ ○ ○
Creative	○ ○ ○ ○ ○

Ratings ☆ ☆ ☆ ☆ ☆

Strain

Grower

Date

Acquired $

Indica   Hybrid   Sativa

☐ Flower   ☐ Edible   ☐ Concentrate

Symptoms Relieved

Notes

Effects	Strength				
Peaceful	○	○	○	○	○
Sleepy	○	○	○	○	○
Pain Relief	○	○	○	○	○
Hungry	○	○	○	○	○
Uplifted	○	○	○	○	○
Creative	○	○	○	○	○

Ratings ☆ ☆ ☆ ☆ ☆

Strain

Grower

Date

Acquired

$

| Indica | Hybrid | Sativa |

☐ Flower   ☐ Edible   ☐ Concentrate

Symptoms Relieved

Sweet
Fruity
Floral
Sour
Spicy
Earthy
Herbal
Woodsy

Notes

Effects	Strength
Peaceful	○ ○ ○ ○ ○
Sleepy	○ ○ ○ ○ ○
Pain Relief	○ ○ ○ ○ ○
Hungry	○ ○ ○ ○ ○
Uplifted	○ ○ ○ ○ ○
Creative	○ ○ ○ ○ ○

Ratings ☆ ☆ ☆ ☆ ☆

Strain

Grower

Date

Acquired

$

| Indica | Hybrid | Sativa |

☐ Flower   ☐ Edible   ☐ Concentrate

Symptoms Relieved

Sweet
Fruity
Floral
Sour
Spicy
Earthy
Herbal
Woodsy

Notes

| Effects | Strength |

Peaceful

Sleepy

Pain Relief

Hungry

Uplifted

Creative

Ratings ☆ ☆ ☆ ☆ ☆

Strain

Grower

Date

Acquired

$

Indica   Hybrid   Sativa

☐ Flower   ☐ Edible   ☐ Concentrate

Symptoms Relieved

Sweet

Fruity   Floral

Sour   Spicy

Earthy   Herbal

Woodsy

Notes

Effects	Strength				
Peaceful	○	○	○	○	○
Sleepy	○	○	○	○	○
Pain Relief	○	○	○	○	○
Hungry	○	○	○	○	○
Uplifted	○	○	○	○	○
Creative	○	○	○	○	○

Ratings ☆ ☆ ☆ ☆ ☆

Strain

Grower

Date

Acquired

$

| Indica | Hybrid | Sativa |

☐ Flower   ☐ Edible   ☐ Concentrate

Symptoms Relieved

Notes

Sweet
Fruity
Floral
Sour
Spicy
Earthy
Herbal
Woodsy

| **Effects** | **Strength** |

Peaceful ○ ○ ○ ○ ○

Sleepy ○ ○ ○ ○ ○

Pain Relief ○ ○ ○ ○ ○

Hungry ○ ○ ○ ○ ○

Uplifted ○ ○ ○ ○ ○

Creative ○ ○ ○ ○ ○

Ratings ☆ ☆ ☆ ☆ ☆

Strain

Grower

Date

Acquired $

| Indica | Hybrid | Sativa |

☐ Flower   ☐ Edible   ☐ Concentrate

Symptoms Relieved

Sweet
Fruity   Floral
Sour   Spicy
Earthy   Herbal
Woodsy

Notes

Effects	**Strength**
Peaceful	○ ○ ○ ○ ○
Sleepy	○ ○ ○ ○ ○
Pain Relief	○ ○ ○ ○ ○
Hungry	○ ○ ○ ○ ○
Uplifted	○ ○ ○ ○ ○
Creative	○ ○ ○ ○ ○

Ratings ☆ ☆ ☆ ☆ ☆

Strain

Grower

Date

Acquired

$

| Indica | Hybrid | Sativa |

☐ Flower   ☐ Edible   ☐ Concentrate

Symptoms Relieved

Sweet

Fruity

Floral

Sour

Spicy

Earthy

Herbal

Woodsy

Notes

Effects	Strength
Peaceful	○ ○ ○ ○ ○
Sleepy	○ ○ ○ ○ ○
Pain Relief	○ ○ ○ ○ ○
Hungry	○ ○ ○ ○ ○
Uplifted	○ ○ ○ ○ ○
Creative	○ ○ ○ ○ ○

Ratings ☆ ☆ ☆ ☆ ☆

Strain

Grower

Date

Acquired

$

| Indica | Hybrid | Sativa |

☐ Flower ☐ Edible ☐ Concentrate

Symptoms Relieved

Notes

Sweet
Fruity
Floral
Sour
Spicy
Earthy
Herbal
Woodsy

Effects	Strength
Peaceful	○ ○ ○ ○ ○
Sleepy	○ ○ ○ ○ ○
Pain Relief	○ ○ ○ ○ ○
Hungry	○ ○ ○ ○ ○
Uplifted	○ ○ ○ ○ ○
Creative	○ ○ ○ ○ ○

Ratings ☆ ☆ ☆ ☆ ☆

Strain

Grower

Date

Acquired

$

| Indica | Hybrid | Sativa |

☐ Flower ☐ Edible ☐ Concentrate

Symptoms Relieved

Sweet

Fruity

Floral

Sour

Spicy

Earthy

Herbal

Woodsy

Notes

Effects	Strength
Peaceful	○ ○ ○ ○ ○
Sleepy	○ ○ ○ ○ ○
Pain Relief	○ ○ ○ ○ ○
Hungry	○ ○ ○ ○ ○
Uplifted	○ ○ ○ ○ ○
Creative	○ ○ ○ ○ ○

Ratings ☆ ☆ ☆ ☆ ☆

Strain

Grower

Date

Acquired

$

| Indica | Hybrid | Sativa |

☐ Flower ☐ Edible ☐ Concentrate

Symptoms Relieved

Notes

Sweet
Fruity
Floral
Sour
Spicy
Earthy
Herbal
Woodsy

Effects	Strength
Peaceful	◯ ◯ ◯ ◯ ◯
Sleepy	◯ ◯ ◯ ◯ ◯
Pain Relief	◯ ◯ ◯ ◯ ◯
Hungry	◯ ◯ ◯ ◯ ◯
Uplifted	◯ ◯ ◯ ◯ ◯
Creative	◯ ◯ ◯ ◯ ◯

Ratings ☆ ☆ ☆ ☆ ☆

Strain

Grower

Date

Acquired

$

| Indica | Hybrid | Sativa |

☐ Flower ☐ Edible ☐ Concentrate

Symptoms Relieved

Sweet

Fruity

Floral

Sour

Spicy

Earthy

Herbal

Woodsy

Notes

Effects	Strength
Peaceful	○ ○ ○ ○ ○
Sleepy	○ ○ ○ ○ ○
Pain Relief	○ ○ ○ ○ ○
Hungry	○ ○ ○ ○ ○
Uplifted	○ ○ ○ ○ ○
Creative	○ ○ ○ ○ ○

Ratings ☆ ☆ ☆ ☆ ☆

Strain

Grower

Date

Acquired

$

| Indica | Hybrid | Sativa |

☐ Flower   ☐ Edible   ☐ Concentrate

Symptoms Relieved

Sweet

Fruity

Floral

Sour

Spicy

Earthy

Herbal

Woodsy

Notes

| **Effects** | **Strength** |

Peaceful	○ ○ ○ ○ ○
Sleepy	○ ○ ○ ○ ○
Pain Relief	○ ○ ○ ○ ○
Hungry	○ ○ ○ ○ ○
Uplifted	○ ○ ○ ○ ○
Creative	○ ○ ○ ○ ○

Ratings ☆ ☆ ☆ ☆ ☆

Strain

Grower

Date

Acquired

$

| Indica | Hybrid | Sativa |

☐ Flower   ☐ Edible   ☐ Concentrate

Symptoms Relieved

Sweet

Fruity

Floral

Sour

Spicy

Earthy

Herbal

Woodsy

Notes

Effects	Strength
Peaceful	○ ○ ○ ○ ○
Sleepy	○ ○ ○ ○ ○
Pain Relief	○ ○ ○ ○ ○
Hungry	○ ○ ○ ○ ○
Uplifted	○ ○ ○ ○ ○
Creative	○ ○ ○ ○ ○

Ratings ☆ ☆ ☆ ☆ ☆

Strain

Grower

Date

Acquired

$

| Indica | Hybrid | Sativa |

☐ Flower   ☐ Edible   ☐ Concentrate

Symptoms Relieved

Sweet

Fruity

Floral

Sour

Spicy

Earthy

Herbal

Woodsy

Notes

Effects	Strength				
Peaceful	○	○	○	○	○
Sleepy	○	○	○	○	○
Pain Relief	○	○	○	○	○
Hungry	○	○	○	○	○
Uplifted	○	○	○	○	○
Creative	○	○	○	○	○

Ratings ☆ ☆ ☆ ☆ ☆

Strain

Grower

Date

Acquired

$

| Indica | Hybrid | Sativa |

☐ Flower ☐ Edible ☐ Concentrate

Symptoms Relieved

Notes

Sweet
Fruity
Floral
Sour
Spicy
Earthy
Herbal
Woodsy

Effects	Strength
Peaceful	○ ○ ○ ○ ○
Sleepy	○ ○ ○ ○ ○
Pain Relief	○ ○ ○ ○ ○
Hungry	○ ○ ○ ○ ○
Uplifted	○ ○ ○ ○ ○
Creative	○ ○ ○ ○ ○

Ratings ☆ ☆ ☆ ☆ ☆

Strain

Grower

Date

Acquired

$

| Indica | Hybrid | Sativa |

☐ Flower   ☐ Edible   ☐ Concentrate

Symptoms Relieved

Sweet

Fruity

Floral

Sour

Spicy

Earthy

Herbal

Woodsy

Notes

Effects	**Strength**
Peaceful	○ ○ ○ ○ ○
Sleepy	○ ○ ○ ○ ○
Pain Relief	○ ○ ○ ○ ○
Hungry	○ ○ ○ ○ ○
Uplifted	○ ○ ○ ○ ○
Creative	○ ○ ○ ○ ○

Ratings ☆ ☆ ☆ ☆ ☆

Strain

Grower

Date

Acquired

$

| Indica | Hybrid | Sativa |

☐ Flower ☐ Edible ☐ Concentrate

Symptoms Relieved

Notes

Effects	Strength
Peaceful	○ ○ ○ ○ ○
Sleepy	○ ○ ○ ○ ○
Pain Relief	○ ○ ○ ○ ○
Hungry	○ ○ ○ ○ ○
Uplifted	○ ○ ○ ○ ○
Creative	○ ○ ○ ○ ○

Ratings ☆ ☆ ☆ ☆ ☆

Strain

Grower

Date

Acquired $

| Indica | Hybrid | Sativa |

☐ Flower   ☐ Edible   ☐ Concentrate

Symptoms Relieved

Sweet

Fruity   Floral

Sour   Spicy

Earthy   Herbal

Woodsy

Notes

Effects	Strength				
Peaceful	○	○	○	○	○
Sleepy	○	○	○	○	○
Pain Relief	○	○	○	○	○
Hungry	○	○	○	○	○
Uplifted	○	○	○	○	○
Creative	○	○	○	○	○

Ratings ☆ ☆ ☆ ☆ ☆

Strain

Grower

Date

Acquired

$

| Indica | Hybrid | Sativa |

☐ Flower   ☐ Edible   ☐ Concentrate

Symptoms Relieved

Sweet

Fruity

Floral

Sour

Spicy

Earthy

Herbal

Woodsy

Notes

| **Effects** | **Strength** |

Peaceful ○ ○ ○ ○ ○

Sleepy ○ ○ ○ ○ ○

Pain Relief ○ ○ ○ ○ ○

Hungry ○ ○ ○ ○ ○

Uplifted ○ ○ ○ ○ ○

Creative ○ ○ ○ ○ ○

Ratings ☆ ☆ ☆ ☆ ☆

Strain

Grower

Date

Acquired

$

Indica	Hybrid	Sativa

☐ Flower   ☐ Edible   ☐ Concentrate

Symptoms Relieved

Notes

Sweet

Fruity

Floral

Sour

Spicy

Earthy

Herbal

Woodsy

Effects	Strength
Peaceful	○ ○ ○ ○ ○
Sleepy	○ ○ ○ ○ ○
Pain Relief	○ ○ ○ ○ ○
Hungry	○ ○ ○ ○ ○
Uplifted	○ ○ ○ ○ ○
Creative	○ ○ ○ ○ ○

Ratings ☆ ☆ ☆ ☆ ☆

Strain

Grower

Date

Acquired

$

| Indica | Hybrid | Sativa |

☐ Flower ☐ Edible ☐ Concentrate

Symptoms Relieved

Sweet
Fruity
Floral
Sour
Spicy
Earthy
Herbal
Woodsy

Notes

Effects	Strength
Peaceful	○ ○ ○ ○ ○
Sleepy	○ ○ ○ ○ ○
Pain Relief	○ ○ ○ ○ ○
Hungry	○ ○ ○ ○ ○
Uplifted	○ ○ ○ ○ ○
Creative	○ ○ ○ ○ ○

Ratings ☆ ☆ ☆ ☆ ☆

Strain

Grower

Date

Acquired

$

| Indica | Hybrid | Sativa |

☐ Flower ☐ Edible ☐ Concentrate

Symptoms Relieved

Sweet

Fruity

Floral

Sour

Spicy

Earthy

Herbal

Woodsy

Notes

Effects	Strength
Peaceful	○ ○ ○ ○ ○
Sleepy	○ ○ ○ ○ ○
Pain Relief	○ ○ ○ ○ ○
Hungry	○ ○ ○ ○ ○
Uplifted	○ ○ ○ ○ ○
Creative	○ ○ ○ ○ ○

Ratings ☆ ☆ ☆ ☆ ☆

Strain

Grower

Date

Acquired

$

| Indica | Hybrid | Sativa |

☐ Flower   ☐ Edible   ☐ Concentrate

Symptoms Relieved

Notes

Effects	**Strength**				
Peaceful	○	○	○	○	○
Sleepy	○	○	○	○	○
Pain Relief	○	○	○	○	○
Hungry	○	○	○	○	○
Uplifted	○	○	○	○	○
Creative	○	○	○	○	○

Ratings ☆ ☆ ☆ ☆ ☆

Strain

Grower

Date

Acquired

$

| Indica | Hybrid | Sativa |

☐ Flower   ☐ Edible   ☐ Concentrate

Symptoms Relieved

Notes

Effects	Strength
Peaceful	○ ○ ○ ○ ○
Sleepy	○ ○ ○ ○ ○
Pain Relief	○ ○ ○ ○ ○
Hungry	○ ○ ○ ○ ○
Uplifted	○ ○ ○ ○ ○
Creative	○ ○ ○ ○ ○

Ratings ☆ ☆ ☆ ☆ ☆

Strain

Grower

Date

Acquired $

| Indica | Hybrid | Sativa |

☐ Flower   ☐ Edible   ☐ Concentrate

Symptoms Relieved

Notes

Sweet
Fruity
Floral
Sour
Spicy
Earthy
Herbal
Woodsy

| **Effects** | **Strength** |

Peaceful ○ ○ ○ ○ ○

Sleepy ○ ○ ○ ○ ○

Pain Relief ○ ○ ○ ○ ○

Hungry ○ ○ ○ ○ ○

Uplifted ○ ○ ○ ○ ○

Creative ○ ○ ○ ○ ○

Ratings ☆ ☆ ☆ ☆ ☆

Strain

Grower

Date

Acquired

$

| Indica | Hybrid | Sativa |

☐ Flower   ☐ Edible   ☐ Concentrate

Symptoms Relieved

Sweet

Fruity

Floral

Sour

Spicy

Earthy

Herbal

Woodsy

Notes

Effects	Strength
Peaceful	○ ○ ○ ○ ○
Sleepy	○ ○ ○ ○ ○
Pain Relief	○ ○ ○ ○ ○
Hungry	○ ○ ○ ○ ○
Uplifted	○ ○ ○ ○ ○
Creative	○ ○ ○ ○ ○

Ratings ☆ ☆ ☆ ☆ ☆

Strain

Grower

Date

Acquired

$

| Indica | Hybrid | Sativa |

☐ Flower   ☐ Edible   ☐ Concentrate

Symptoms Relieved

Notes

Sweet

Fruity

Floral

Sour

Spicy

Earthy

Herbal

Woodsy

Effects	Strength
Peaceful	○ ○ ○ ○ ○
Sleepy	○ ○ ○ ○ ○
Pain Relief	○ ○ ○ ○ ○
Hungry	○ ○ ○ ○ ○
Uplifted	○ ○ ○ ○ ○
Creative	○ ○ ○ ○ ○

Ratings ☆ ☆ ☆ ☆ ☆

Strain

Grower

Date

Acquired

$

| Indica | Hybrid | Sativa |

☐ Flower   ☐ Edible   ☐ Concentrate

Symptoms Relieved

Sweet

Fruity

Floral

Sour

Spicy

Earthy

Herbal

Woodsy

Notes

Effects	**Strength**
Peaceful	○ ○ ○ ○ ○
Sleepy	○ ○ ○ ○ ○
Pain Relief	○ ○ ○ ○ ○
Hungry	○ ○ ○ ○ ○
Uplifted	○ ○ ○ ○ ○
Creative	○ ○ ○ ○ ○

Ratings ☆ ☆ ☆ ☆ ☆

Strain

Grower

Date

Acquired $

| Indica | Hybrid | Sativa |

☐ Flower   ☐ Edible   ☐ Concentrate

Symptoms Relieved

Sweet
Fruity   Floral
Sour   Spicy
Earthy   Herbal
Woodsy

Notes

Effects	Strength
Peaceful	○ ○ ○ ○ ○
Sleepy	○ ○ ○ ○ ○
Pain Relief	○ ○ ○ ○ ○
Hungry	○ ○ ○ ○ ○
Uplifted	○ ○ ○ ○ ○
Creative	○ ○ ○ ○ ○

Ratings ☆ ☆ ☆ ☆ ☆

Strain

Grower

Date

Acquired

$

| Indica | Hybrid | Sativa |

☐ Flower ☐ Edible ☐ Concentrate

Symptoms Relieved

Notes

Effects	Strength
Peaceful	○ ○ ○ ○ ○
Sleepy	○ ○ ○ ○ ○
Pain Relief	○ ○ ○ ○ ○
Hungry	○ ○ ○ ○ ○
Uplifted	○ ○ ○ ○ ○
Creative	○ ○ ○ ○ ○

Ratings ☆ ☆ ☆ ☆ ☆

Strain

Grower

Date

Acquired

$

| Indica | Hybrid | Sativa |

☐ Flower   ☐ Edible   ☐ Concentrate

Symptoms Relieved

Sweet
Fruity
Floral
Sour
Spicy
Earthy
Herbal
Woodsy

Notes

Effects	**Strength**
Peaceful	○ ○ ○ ○ ○
Sleepy	○ ○ ○ ○ ○
Pain Relief	○ ○ ○ ○ ○
Hungry	○ ○ ○ ○ ○
Uplifted	○ ○ ○ ○ ○
Creative	○ ○ ○ ○ ○

Ratings ☆ ☆ ☆ ☆ ☆

Strain

Grower

Date

Acquired $

| Indica | Hybrid | Sativa |

☐ Flower   ☐ Edible   ☐ Concentrate

Symptoms Relieved

Sweet
Fruity — Floral
Sour — Spicy
Earthy — Herbal
Woodsy

Notes

Effects	**Strength**				
Peaceful	○	○	○	○	○
Sleepy	○	○	○	○	○
Pain Relief	○	○	○	○	○
Hungry	○	○	○	○	○
Uplifted	○	○	○	○	○
Creative	○	○	○	○	○

Ratings ☆ ☆ ☆ ☆ ☆

Strain

Grower

Date

Acquired

$

| Indica | Hybrid | Sativa |

☐ Flower   ☐ Edible   ☐ Concentrate

Symptoms Relieved

Sweet
Fruity
Floral
Sour
Spicy
Earthy
Herbal
Woodsy

Notes

Effects	Strength
Peaceful	○ ○ ○ ○ ○
Sleepy	○ ○ ○ ○ ○
Pain Relief	○ ○ ○ ○ ○
Hungry	○ ○ ○ ○ ○
Uplifted	○ ○ ○ ○ ○
Creative	○ ○ ○ ○ ○

Ratings ☆ ☆ ☆ ☆ ☆

Strain

Grower

Date

Acquired

$

| Indica | Hybrid | Sativa |

☐ Flower   ☐ Edible   ☐ Concentrate

Symptoms Relieved

Sweet

Fruity

Floral

Sour

Spicy

Earthy

Herbal

Woodsy

Notes

Effects	Strength				
Peaceful	○	○	○	○	○
Sleepy	○	○	○	○	○
Pain Relief	○	○	○	○	○
Hungry	○	○	○	○	○
Uplifted	○	○	○	○	○
Creative	○	○	○	○	○

Ratings ☆ ☆ ☆ ☆ ☆

Strain

Grower

Date

Acquired

$

| Indica | Hybrid | Sativa |

☐ Flower ☐ Edible ☐ Concentrate

Symptoms Relieved

Sweet
Fruity   Floral

Sour   Spicy

Earthy   Herbal
Woodsy

Notes

Effects	**Strength**
Peaceful	◯ ◯ ◯ ◯ ◯
Sleepy	◯ ◯ ◯ ◯ ◯
Pain Relief	◯ ◯ ◯ ◯ ◯
Hungry	◯ ◯ ◯ ◯ ◯
Uplifted	◯ ◯ ◯ ◯ ◯
Creative	◯ ◯ ◯ ◯ ◯

Ratings ☆ ☆ ☆ ☆ ☆

Strain

Grower

Date

Acquired

$

| Indica | Hybrid | Sativa |

☐ Flower   ☐ Edible   ☐ Concentrate

Symptoms Relieved

Notes

Effects	Strength
Peaceful	○ ○ ○ ○ ○
Sleepy	○ ○ ○ ○ ○
Pain Relief	○ ○ ○ ○ ○
Hungry	○ ○ ○ ○ ○
Uplifted	○ ○ ○ ○ ○
Creative	○ ○ ○ ○ ○

Ratings ☆ ☆ ☆ ☆ ☆

Strain

Grower

Date

Acquired

$

| Indica | Hybrid | Sativa |

☐ Flower   ☐ Edible   ☐ Concentrate

Symptoms Relieved

Sweet
Fruity
Floral
Sour
Spicy
Earthy
Herbal
Woodsy

Notes

| **Effects** | **Strength** |

Peaceful ○ ○ ○ ○ ○

Sleepy ○ ○ ○ ○ ○

Pain Relief ○ ○ ○ ○ ○

Hungry ○ ○ ○ ○ ○

Uplifted ○ ○ ○ ○ ○

Creative ○ ○ ○ ○ ○

Ratings ☆ ☆ ☆ ☆ ☆

Strain

Grower

Date

Acquired

$

| Indica | Hybrid | Sativa |

☐ Flower ☐ Edible ☐ Concentrate

Symptoms Relieved

Sweet
Fruity
Floral
Sour
Spicy
Earthy
Herbal
Woodsy

Notes

Effects	Strength
Peaceful	○ ○ ○ ○ ○
Sleepy	○ ○ ○ ○ ○
Pain Relief	○ ○ ○ ○ ○
Hungry	○ ○ ○ ○ ○
Uplifted	○ ○ ○ ○ ○
Creative	○ ○ ○ ○ ○

Ratings ☆ ☆ ☆ ☆ ☆

Strain

Grower

Date

Acquired

$

| Indica | Hybrid | Sativa |

☐ Flower ☐ Edible ☐ Concentrate

Symptoms Relieved

Notes

Sweet

Fruity

Floral

Sour

Spicy

Earthy

Herbal

Woodsy

Effects	Strength
Peaceful	○ ○ ○ ○ ○
Sleepy	○ ○ ○ ○ ○
Pain Relief	○ ○ ○ ○ ○
Hungry	○ ○ ○ ○ ○
Uplifted	○ ○ ○ ○ ○
Creative	○ ○ ○ ○ ○

Ratings ☆ ☆ ☆ ☆ ☆

Strain

Grower

Date

Acquired

$

| Indica | Hybrid | Sativa |

☐ Flower   ☐ Edible   ☐ Concentrate

Symptoms Relieved

Notes

Sweet

Fruity

Floral

Sour

Spicy

Earthy

Herbal

Woodsy

Effects	Strength
Peaceful	○ ○ ○ ○ ○
Sleepy	○ ○ ○ ○ ○
Pain Relief	○ ○ ○ ○ ○
Hungry	○ ○ ○ ○ ○
Uplifted	○ ○ ○ ○ ○
Creative	○ ○ ○ ○ ○

Ratings ☆ ☆ ☆ ☆ ☆

Strain

Grower

Date

Acquired $

| Indica | Hybrid | Sativa |

☐ Flower   ☐ Edible   ☐ Concentrate

Symptoms Relieved

Flavor Wheel: Sweet, Floral, Spicy, Herbal, Woodsy, Earthy, Sour, Fruity

Notes

Effects	Strength				
Peaceful	○	○	○	○	○
Sleepy	○	○	○	○	○
Pain Relief	○	○	○	○	○
Hungry	○	○	○	○	○
Uplifted	○	○	○	○	○
Creative	○	○	○	○	○

Ratings ☆ ☆ ☆ ☆ ☆

Strain

Grower

Date

Acquired

$

| Indica | Hybrid | Sativa |

☐ Flower   ☐ Edible   ☐ Concentrate

Symptoms Relieved

Sweet

Fruity

Floral

Sour

Spicy

Earthy

Herbal

Woodsy

Notes

Effects	Strength
Peaceful	○ ○ ○ ○ ○
Sleepy	○ ○ ○ ○ ○
Pain Relief	○ ○ ○ ○ ○
Hungry	○ ○ ○ ○ ○
Uplifted	○ ○ ○ ○ ○
Creative	○ ○ ○ ○ ○

Ratings ☆ ☆ ☆ ☆ ☆

Strain

Grower

Date

Acquired

$

| Indica | Hybrid | Sativa |

☐ Flower   ☐ Edible   ☐ Concentrate

Symptoms Relieved

Notes

Sweet
Fruity
Floral
Sour
Spicy
Earthy
Herbal
Woodsy

| **Effects** | **Strength** |

Peaceful

Sleepy

Pain Relief

Hungry

Uplifted

Creative

Ratings ☆ ☆ ☆ ☆ ☆

Strain

Grower

Date

Acquired

$

| Indica | Hybrid | Sativa |

☐ Flower ☐ Edible ☐ Concentrate

Symptoms Relieved

Sweet

Fruity

Floral

Sour

Spicy

Earthy

Herbal

Woodsy

Notes

Effects	**Strength**
Peaceful	○ ○ ○ ○ ○
Sleepy	○ ○ ○ ○ ○
Pain Relief	○ ○ ○ ○ ○
Hungry	○ ○ ○ ○ ○
Uplifted	○ ○ ○ ○ ○
Creative	○ ○ ○ ○ ○

Ratings ☆ ☆ ☆ ☆ ☆

Strain

Grower

Date

Acquired

$

| Indica | Hybrid | Sativa |

☐ Flower   ☐ Edible   ☐ Concentrate

Symptoms Relieved

Notes

Effects	**Strength**
Peaceful	○ ○ ○ ○ ○
Sleepy	○ ○ ○ ○ ○
Pain Relief	○ ○ ○ ○ ○
Hungry	○ ○ ○ ○ ○
Uplifted	○ ○ ○ ○ ○
Creative	○ ○ ○ ○ ○

Ratings ☆ ☆ ☆ ☆ ☆

Strain

Grower

Date

Acquired

$

| Indica | Hybrid | Sativa |

☐ Flower   ☐ Edible   ☐ Concentrate

Symptoms Relieved

Notes

Effects	Strength
Peaceful	○ ○ ○ ○ ○
Sleepy	○ ○ ○ ○ ○
Pain Relief	○ ○ ○ ○ ○
Hungry	○ ○ ○ ○ ○
Uplifted	○ ○ ○ ○ ○
Creative	○ ○ ○ ○ ○

Ratings ☆ ☆ ☆ ☆ ☆

Strain

Grower

Date

Acquired $

| Indica | Hybrid | Sativa |

☐ Flower ☐ Edible ☐ Concentrate

Symptoms Relieved

Notes

Sweet
Fruity
Floral
Sour
Spicy
Earthy
Herbal
Woodsy

Effects	**Strength**
Peaceful	○ ○ ○ ○ ○
Sleepy	○ ○ ○ ○ ○
Pain Relief	○ ○ ○ ○ ○
Hungry	○ ○ ○ ○ ○
Uplifted	○ ○ ○ ○ ○
Creative	○ ○ ○ ○ ○

Ratings ☆ ☆ ☆ ☆ ☆

Strain

Grower

Date

Acquired

$

| Indica | Hybrid | Sativa |

☐ Flower   ☐ Edible   ☐ Concentrate

Symptoms Relieved

Notes

Sweet
Fruity
Floral
Sour
Spicy
Earthy
Herbal
Woodsy

Effects	**Strength**
Peaceful	○ ○ ○ ○ ○
Sleepy	○ ○ ○ ○ ○
Pain Relief	○ ○ ○ ○ ○
Hungry	○ ○ ○ ○ ○
Uplifted	○ ○ ○ ○ ○
Creative	○ ○ ○ ○ ○

Ratings ☆ ☆ ☆ ☆ ☆

Strain

Grower

Date

Acquired

$

| Indica | Hybrid | Sativa |

☐ Flower   ☐ Edible   ☐ Concentrate

Symptoms Relieved

Sweet
Fruity
Floral
Sour
Spicy
Earthy
Herbal
Woodsy

Notes

Effects	Strength				
Peaceful	○	○	○	○	○
Sleepy	○	○	○	○	○
Pain Relief	○	○	○	○	○
Hungry	○	○	○	○	○
Uplifted	○	○	○	○	○
Creative	○	○	○	○	○

Ratings ☆ ☆ ☆ ☆ ☆

Strain

Grower

Date

Acquired

$

| Indica | Hybrid | Sativa |

☐ Flower ☐ Edible ☐ Concentrate

Symptoms Relieved

Sweet
Fruity
Floral
Sour
Spicy
Earthy
Herbal
Woodsy

Notes

Effects	Strength
Peaceful	○ ○ ○ ○ ○
Sleepy	○ ○ ○ ○ ○
Pain Relief	○ ○ ○ ○ ○
Hungry	○ ○ ○ ○ ○
Uplifted	○ ○ ○ ○ ○
Creative	○ ○ ○ ○ ○

Ratings ☆ ☆ ☆ ☆ ☆

Strain

Grower

Date

Acquired

$

| Indica | Hybrid | Sativa |

☐ Flower ☐ Edible ☐ Concentrate

Symptoms Relieved

Notes

Sweet
Fruity
Floral
Sour
Spicy
Earthy
Herbal
Woodsy

Effects	Strength
Peaceful	○ ○ ○ ○ ○
Sleepy	○ ○ ○ ○ ○
Pain Relief	○ ○ ○ ○ ○
Hungry	○ ○ ○ ○ ○
Uplifted	○ ○ ○ ○ ○
Creative	○ ○ ○ ○ ○

Ratings ☆ ☆ ☆ ☆ ☆

Strain

Grower

Date

Acquired

$

| Indica | Hybrid | Sativa |

☐ Flower   ☐ Edible   ☐ Concentrate

Symptoms Relieved

Sweet

Fruity

Floral

Sour

Spicy

Earthy

Herbal

Woodsy

Notes

| **Effects** | **Strength** |

Peaceful   ○ ○ ○ ○ ○

Sleepy   ○ ○ ○ ○ ○

Pain Relief   ○ ○ ○ ○ ○

Hungry   ○ ○ ○ ○ ○

Uplifted   ○ ○ ○ ○ ○

Creative   ○ ○ ○ ○ ○

Ratings ☆ ☆ ☆ ☆ ☆

Strain

Grower

Date

Acquired

$

| Indica | Hybrid | Sativa |

☐ Flower ☐ Edible ☐ Concentrate

Symptoms Relieved

Sweet
Fruity
Floral
Sour
Spicy
Earthy
Herbal
Woodsy

Notes

Effects	Strength
Peaceful	○ ○ ○ ○ ○
Sleepy	○ ○ ○ ○ ○
Pain Relief	○ ○ ○ ○ ○
Hungry	○ ○ ○ ○ ○
Uplifted	○ ○ ○ ○ ○
Creative	○ ○ ○ ○ ○

Ratings ☆ ☆ ☆ ☆ ☆

Strain

Grower

Date

Acquired

$

| Indica | Hybrid | Sativa |

☐ Flower ☐ Edible ☐ Concentrate

Symptoms Relieved

Notes

Sweet

Fruity

Floral

Sour

Spicy

Earthy

Herbal

Woodsy

Effects	Strength
Peaceful	○ ○ ○ ○ ○
Sleepy	○ ○ ○ ○ ○
Pain Relief	○ ○ ○ ○ ○
Hungry	○ ○ ○ ○ ○
Uplifted	○ ○ ○ ○ ○
Creative	○ ○ ○ ○ ○

Ratings ☆ ☆ ☆ ☆ ☆

Strain

Grower

Date

Acquired

$

| Indica | Hybrid | Sativa |

☐ Flower ☐ Edible ☐ Concentrate

Symptoms Relieved

Sweet

Fruity

Floral

Sour

Spicy

Earthy

Herbal

Woodsy

Notes

Effects	Strength
Peaceful	○ ○ ○ ○ ○
Sleepy	○ ○ ○ ○ ○
Pain Relief	○ ○ ○ ○ ○
Hungry	○ ○ ○ ○ ○
Uplifted	○ ○ ○ ○ ○
Creative	○ ○ ○ ○ ○

Ratings ☆ ☆ ☆ ☆ ☆

Strain

Grower

Date

Acquired $

| Indica | Hybrid | Sativa |

☐ Flower   ☐ Edible   ☐ Concentrate

Symptoms Relieved

Notes

Sweet
Fruity
Floral
Sour
Spicy
Earthy
Herbal
Woodsy

Effects	Strength
Peaceful	○ ○ ○ ○ ○
Sleepy	○ ○ ○ ○ ○
Pain Relief	○ ○ ○ ○ ○
Hungry	○ ○ ○ ○ ○
Uplifted	○ ○ ○ ○ ○
Creative	○ ○ ○ ○ ○

Ratings ☆ ☆ ☆ ☆ ☆

Strain

Grower

Date

Acquired $

| Indica | Hybrid | Sativa |

☐ Flower   ☐ Edible   ☐ Concentrate

Symptoms Relieved

Notes

Sweet
Fruity   Floral
Sour   Spicy
Earthy   Herbal
Woodsy

Effects	Strength
Peaceful	○ ○ ○ ○ ○
Sleepy	○ ○ ○ ○ ○
Pain Relief	○ ○ ○ ○ ○
Hungry	○ ○ ○ ○ ○
Uplifted	○ ○ ○ ○ ○
Creative	○ ○ ○ ○ ○

Ratings ☆ ☆ ☆ ☆ ☆

Strain

Grower

Date

Acquired

$

| Indica | Hybrid | Sativa |

☐ Flower   ☐ Edible   ☐ Concentrate

Symptoms Relieved

Notes

Effects	Strength
Peaceful	○ ○ ○ ○ ○
Sleepy	○ ○ ○ ○ ○
Pain Relief	○ ○ ○ ○ ○
Hungry	○ ○ ○ ○ ○
Uplifted	○ ○ ○ ○ ○
Creative	○ ○ ○ ○ ○

Ratings ☆ ☆ ☆ ☆ ☆

Strain

Grower

Date

Acquired

$

| Indica | Hybrid | Sativa |

☐ Flower ☐ Edible ☐ Concentrate

Symptoms Relieved

Notes

Sweet
Fruity
Floral
Sour
Spicy
Earthy
Herbal
Woodsy

Effects	**Strength**
Peaceful	○ ○ ○ ○ ○
Sleepy	○ ○ ○ ○ ○
Pain Relief	○ ○ ○ ○ ○
Hungry	○ ○ ○ ○ ○
Uplifted	○ ○ ○ ○ ○
Creative	○ ○ ○ ○ ○

Ratings ☆ ☆ ☆ ☆ ☆

Strain

Grower

Date

Acquired

$

| Indica | Hybrid | Sativa |

☐ Flower   ☐ Edible   ☐ Concentrate

Symptoms Relieved

Sweet

Fruity

Floral

Sour

Spicy

Earthy

Herbal

Woodsy

Notes

Effects	**Strength**
Peaceful	○ ○ ○ ○ ○
Sleepy	○ ○ ○ ○ ○
Pain Relief	○ ○ ○ ○ ○
Hungry	○ ○ ○ ○ ○
Uplifted	○ ○ ○ ○ ○
Creative	○ ○ ○ ○ ○

Ratings ☆ ☆ ☆ ☆ ☆

Strain

Grower ______________________

Acquired ______________________

Date ______________________

$ ______________________

| Indica | Hybrid | Sativa |

☐ Flower ☐ Edible ☐ Concentrate

Symptoms Relieved

____
____
____
____

Sweet
Fruity
Floral
Sour
Spicy
Earthy
Herbal
Woodsy

Notes

____
____
____
____
____
____
____

Effects	Strength
Peaceful	○ ○ ○ ○ ○
Sleepy	○ ○ ○ ○ ○
Pain Relief	○ ○ ○ ○ ○
Hungry	○ ○ ○ ○ ○
Uplifted	○ ○ ○ ○ ○
Creative	○ ○ ○ ○ ○

Ratings ☆ ☆ ☆ ☆ ☆

Strain

Grower

Date

Acquired

$

| Indica | Hybrid | Sativa |

☐ Flower ☐ Edible ☐ Concentrate

Symptoms Relieved

Notes

Effects	Strength
Peaceful	○ ○ ○ ○ ○
Sleepy	○ ○ ○ ○ ○
Pain Relief	○ ○ ○ ○ ○
Hungry	○ ○ ○ ○ ○
Uplifted	○ ○ ○ ○ ○
Creative	○ ○ ○ ○ ○

Ratings ☆ ☆ ☆ ☆ ☆

Strain

Grower ___________________

Date ___________________

Acquired ___________________

$ ___________________

| Indica | Hybrid | Sativa |

☐ Flower ☐ Edible ☐ Concentrate

Symptoms Relieved

____
____
____
____
____

Notes

____
____
____
____
____
____
____
____

Effects	Strength
Peaceful	◯ ◯ ◯ ◯ ◯
Sleepy	◯ ◯ ◯ ◯ ◯
Pain Relief	◯ ◯ ◯ ◯ ◯
Hungry	◯ ◯ ◯ ◯ ◯
Uplifted	◯ ◯ ◯ ◯ ◯
Creative	◯ ◯ ◯ ◯ ◯

Ratings ☆ ☆ ☆ ☆ ☆

Strain

Grower

Date

Acquired

$

| Indica | Hybrid | Sativa |

☐ Flower   ☐ Edible   ☐ Concentrate

Symptoms Relieved

Notes

Effects	Strength
Peaceful	○ ○ ○ ○ ○
Sleepy	○ ○ ○ ○ ○
Pain Relief	○ ○ ○ ○ ○
Hungry	○ ○ ○ ○ ○
Uplifted	○ ○ ○ ○ ○
Creative	○ ○ ○ ○ ○

Ratings ☆ ☆ ☆ ☆ ☆

Strain

Grower

Date

Acquired

$

| Indica | Hybrid | Sativa |

☐ Flower ☐ Edible ☐ Concentrate

Symptoms Relieved

Sweet
Fruity
Floral
Sour
Spicy
Earthy
Herbal
Woodsy

Notes

Effects	Strength
Peaceful	○ ○ ○ ○ ○
Sleepy	○ ○ ○ ○ ○
Pain Relief	○ ○ ○ ○ ○
Hungry	○ ○ ○ ○ ○
Uplifted	○ ○ ○ ○ ○
Creative	○ ○ ○ ○ ○

Ratings ☆ ☆ ☆ ☆ ☆

Strain

Grower

Date

Acquired

$

| Indica | Hybrid | Sativa |

☐ Flower   ☐ Edible   ☐ Concentrate

Symptoms Relieved

Sweet

Fruity

Floral

Sour

Spicy

Earthy

Herbal

Woodsy

Notes

Effects	**Strength**				
Peaceful	○	○	○	○	○
Sleepy	○	○	○	○	○
Pain Relief	○	○	○	○	○
Hungry	○	○	○	○	○
Uplifted	○	○	○	○	○
Creative	○	○	○	○	○

Ratings ☆ ☆ ☆ ☆ ☆

Strain

Grower

Date

Acquired

$

| Indica | Hybrid | Sativa |

☐ Flower　　☐ Edible　　☐ Concentrate

Symptoms Relieved

Sweet

Fruity

Floral

Sour

Spicy

Earthy

Herbal

Woodsy

Notes

Effects	Strength
Peaceful	○ ○ ○ ○ ○
Sleepy	○ ○ ○ ○ ○
Pain Relief	○ ○ ○ ○ ○
Hungry	○ ○ ○ ○ ○
Uplifted	○ ○ ○ ○ ○
Creative	○ ○ ○ ○ ○

Ratings ☆ ☆ ☆ ☆ ☆

Strain

Grower

Date

Acquired

$

| Indica | Hybrid | Sativa |

☐ Flower   ☐ Edible   ☐ Concentrate

Symptoms Relieved

Sweet
Fruity
Floral
Sour
Spicy
Earthy
Herbal
Woodsy

Notes

Effects	Strength
Peaceful	○ ○ ○ ○ ○
Sleepy	○ ○ ○ ○ ○
Pain Relief	○ ○ ○ ○ ○
Hungry	○ ○ ○ ○ ○
Uplifted	○ ○ ○ ○ ○
Creative	○ ○ ○ ○ ○

Ratings ☆ ☆ ☆ ☆ ☆

Strain

Grower

Date

Acquired $

| |
| Indica   Hybrid   Sativa |

☐ Flower   ☐ Edible   ☐ Concentrate

Symptoms Relieved

Sweet
Fruity   Floral

Sour   Spicy

Earthy   Herbal
Woodsy

Notes

Effects	Strength
Peaceful	○ ○ ○ ○ ○
Sleepy	○ ○ ○ ○ ○
Pain Relief	○ ○ ○ ○ ○
Hungry	○ ○ ○ ○ ○
Uplifted	○ ○ ○ ○ ○
Creative	○ ○ ○ ○ ○

Ratings ☆ ☆ ☆ ☆ ☆

Strain

Grower

Date

Acquired $

| Indica | Hybrid | Sativa |

☐ Flower ☐ Edible ☐ Concentrate

Symptoms Relieved

Sweet
Fruity
Floral
Sour
Spicy
Earthy
Herbal
Woodsy

Notes

Effects	Strength
Peaceful	○ ○ ○ ○ ○
Sleepy	○ ○ ○ ○ ○
Pain Relief	○ ○ ○ ○ ○
Hungry	○ ○ ○ ○ ○
Uplifted	○ ○ ○ ○ ○
Creative	○ ○ ○ ○ ○

Ratings ☆ ☆ ☆ ☆ ☆

Strain

Grower

Date

Acquired

$

| Indica | Hybrid | Sativa |

☐ Flower　　☐ Edible　　☐ Concentrate

Symptoms Relieved

Sweet
Fruity
Floral
Sour
Spicy
Earthy
Herbal
Woodsy

Notes

Effects	Strength
Peaceful	○ ○ ○ ○ ○
Sleepy	○ ○ ○ ○ ○
Pain Relief	○ ○ ○ ○ ○
Hungry	○ ○ ○ ○ ○
Uplifted	○ ○ ○ ○ ○
Creative	○ ○ ○ ○ ○

Ratings　☆ ☆ ☆ ☆ ☆

Strain

Grower

Date

Acquired

$

| Indica | Hybrid | Sativa |

☐ Flower   ☐ Edible   ☐ Concentrate

Symptoms Relieved

Sweet

Fruity

Floral

Sour

Spicy

Earthy

Herbal

Woodsy

Notes

Effects	Strength
Peaceful	○ ○ ○ ○ ○
Sleepy	○ ○ ○ ○ ○
Pain Relief	○ ○ ○ ○ ○
Hungry	○ ○ ○ ○ ○
Uplifted	○ ○ ○ ○ ○
Creative	○ ○ ○ ○ ○

Ratings ☆ ☆ ☆ ☆ ☆

Strain

Grower

Date

Acquired

$

| Indica | Hybrid | Sativa |

☐ Flower　　☐ Edible　　☐ Concentrate

Symptoms Relieved

Notes

Effects	**Strength**
Peaceful	○ ○ ○ ○ ○
Sleepy	○ ○ ○ ○ ○
Pain Relief	○ ○ ○ ○ ○
Hungry	○ ○ ○ ○ ○
Uplifted	○ ○ ○ ○ ○
Creative	○ ○ ○ ○ ○

Ratings ☆ ☆ ☆ ☆ ☆

Strain

Grower

Date

Acquired

$

| Indica | Hybrid | Sativa |

☐ Flower   ☐ Edible   ☐ Concentrate

Symptoms Relieved

Notes

Sweet

Fruity

Floral

Sour

Spicy

Earthy

Herbal

Woodsy

Effects	Strength
Peaceful	○ ○ ○ ○ ○
Sleepy	○ ○ ○ ○ ○
Pain Relief	○ ○ ○ ○ ○
Hungry	○ ○ ○ ○ ○
Uplifted	○ ○ ○ ○ ○
Creative	○ ○ ○ ○ ○

Ratings ☆ ☆ ☆ ☆ ☆

Strain

Grower

Date

Acquired

$

| Indica | Hybrid | Sativa |

☐ Flower   ☐ Edible   ☐ Concentrate

Symptoms Relieved

Notes

Sweet
Fruity
Floral
Sour
Spicy
Earthy
Herbal
Woodsy

Effects	Strength
Peaceful	○ ○ ○ ○ ○
Sleepy	○ ○ ○ ○ ○
Pain Relief	○ ○ ○ ○ ○
Hungry	○ ○ ○ ○ ○
Uplifted	○ ○ ○ ○ ○
Creative	○ ○ ○ ○ ○

Ratings ☆ ☆ ☆ ☆ ☆

Strain

Grower

Date

Acquired

$

| Indica | Hybrid | Sativa |

☐ Flower   ☐ Edible   ☐ Concentrate

Symptoms Relieved

Notes

Effects	Strength
Peaceful	○ ○ ○ ○ ○
Sleepy	○ ○ ○ ○ ○
Pain Relief	○ ○ ○ ○ ○
Hungry	○ ○ ○ ○ ○
Uplifted	○ ○ ○ ○ ○
Creative	○ ○ ○ ○ ○

Ratings ☆ ☆ ☆ ☆ ☆

Strain

Grower

Date

Acquired

$

| Indica | Hybrid | Sativa |

☐ Flower   ☐ Edible   ☐ Concentrate

Symptoms Relieved

Sweet
Fruity
Floral
Sour
Spicy
Earthy
Herbal
Woodsy

Notes

| Effects | Strength |

Peaceful ○ ○ ○ ○ ○

Sleepy ○ ○ ○ ○ ○

Pain Relief ○ ○ ○ ○ ○

Hungry ○ ○ ○ ○ ○

Uplifted ○ ○ ○ ○ ○

Creative ○ ○ ○ ○ ○

Ratings ☆ ☆ ☆ ☆ ☆

Strain

Grower

Date

Acquired

$

| Indica | Hybrid | Sativa |

☐ Flower   ☐ Edible   ☐ Concentrate

Symptoms Relieved

Sweet

Fruity

Floral

Sour

Spicy

Earthy

Herbal

Woodsy

Notes

Effects	Strength
Peaceful	○ ○ ○ ○ ○
Sleepy	○ ○ ○ ○ ○
Pain Relief	○ ○ ○ ○ ○
Hungry	○ ○ ○ ○ ○
Uplifted	○ ○ ○ ○ ○
Creative	○ ○ ○ ○ ○

Ratings ☆ ☆ ☆ ☆ ☆

Strain

Grower

Date

Acquired

$

| Indica | Hybrid | Sativa |

☐ Flower   ☐ Edible   ☐ Concentrate

Symptoms Relieved

Sweet

Fruity

Floral

Sour

Spicy

Earthy

Herbal

Woodsy

Notes

Effects   **Strength**

Peaceful   ○ ○ ○ ○ ○

Sleepy   ○ ○ ○ ○ ○

Pain Relief   ○ ○ ○ ○ ○

Hungry   ○ ○ ○ ○ ○

Uplifted   ○ ○ ○ ○ ○

Creative   ○ ○ ○ ○ ○

Ratings   ☆ ☆ ☆ ☆ ☆

Strain

Grower

Date

Acquired

$

| Indica | Hybrid | Sativa |

☐ Flower   ☐ Edible   ☐ Concentrate

Symptoms Relieved

Notes

Sweet

Fruity

Floral

Sour

Spicy

Earthy

Herbal

Woodsy

| **Effects** | **Strength** |

Peaceful ○ ○ ○ ○ ○

Sleepy ○ ○ ○ ○ ○

Pain Relief ○ ○ ○ ○ ○

Hungry ○ ○ ○ ○ ○

Uplifted ○ ○ ○ ○ ○

Creative ○ ○ ○ ○ ○

Ratings ☆ ☆ ☆ ☆ ☆

Strain

Grower

Date

Acquired $

| Indica | Hybrid | Sativa |

☐ Flower   ☐ Edible   ☐ Concentrate

Symptoms Relieved

Notes

| **Effects** | **Strength** |

Peaceful ○ ○ ○ ○ ○

Sleepy ○ ○ ○ ○ ○

Pain Relief ○ ○ ○ ○ ○

Hungry ○ ○ ○ ○ ○

Uplifted ○ ○ ○ ○ ○

Creative ○ ○ ○ ○ ○

Ratings ☆ ☆ ☆ ☆ ☆

Strain

Grower

Date

Acquired

$

| Indica | Hybrid | Sativa |

☐ Flower   ☐ Edible   ☐ Concentrate

Symptoms Relieved

Notes

Sweet

Fruity

Floral

Sour

Spicy

Earthy

Herbal

Woodsy

Effects	Strength
Peaceful	○ ○ ○ ○ ○
Sleepy	○ ○ ○ ○ ○
Pain Relief	○ ○ ○ ○ ○
Hungry	○ ○ ○ ○ ○
Uplifted	○ ○ ○ ○ ○
Creative	○ ○ ○ ○ ○

Ratings ☆ ☆ ☆ ☆ ☆

Strain

Grower

Date

Acquired

$

| Indica | Hybrid | Sativa |

☐ Flower   ☐ Edible   ☐ Concentrate

Symptoms Relieved

Sweet
Fruity
Floral
Sour
Spicy
Earthy
Herbal
Woodsy

Notes

Effects	Strength
Peaceful	○ ○ ○ ○ ○
Sleepy	○ ○ ○ ○ ○
Pain Relief	○ ○ ○ ○ ○
Hungry	○ ○ ○ ○ ○
Uplifted	○ ○ ○ ○ ○
Creative	○ ○ ○ ○ ○

Ratings ☆ ☆ ☆ ☆ ☆

Strain

Grower

Date

Acquired $

| Indica | Hybrid | Sativa |

☐ Flower   ☐ Edible   ☐ Concentrate

Symptoms Relieved

Notes

Effects	Strength
Peaceful	○ ○ ○ ○ ○
Sleepy	○ ○ ○ ○ ○
Pain Relief	○ ○ ○ ○ ○
Hungry	○ ○ ○ ○ ○
Uplifted	○ ○ ○ ○ ○
Creative	○ ○ ○ ○ ○

Ratings ☆ ☆ ☆ ☆ ☆

Strain

Grower

Date

Acquired $

| Indica | Hybrid | Sativa |

☐ Flower   ☐ Edible   ☐ Concentrate

Symptoms Relieved

Sweet
Fruity   Floral
Sour   Spicy
Earthy   Herbal
Woodsy

Notes

Effects	Strength
Peaceful	○ ○ ○ ○ ○
Sleepy	○ ○ ○ ○ ○
Pain Relief	○ ○ ○ ○ ○
Hungry	○ ○ ○ ○ ○
Uplifted	○ ○ ○ ○ ○
Creative	○ ○ ○ ○ ○

Ratings ☆ ☆ ☆ ☆ ☆

Strain

Grower

Date

Acquired

$

Indica	Hybrid	Sativa

- [ ] Flower
- [ ] Edible
- [ ] Concentrate

Symptoms Relieved

Notes

Effects	Strength				
Peaceful	○	○	○	○	○
Sleepy	○	○	○	○	○
Pain Relief	○	○	○	○	○
Hungry	○	○	○	○	○
Uplifted	○	○	○	○	○
Creative	○	○	○	○	○

Ratings ☆ ☆ ☆ ☆ ☆

Strain

Grower

Date

Acquired

$

| Indica | Hybrid | Sativa |

☐ Flower   ☐ Edible   ☐ Concentrate

Symptoms Relieved

Notes

Sweet
Fruity
Floral
Sour
Spicy
Earthy
Herbal
Woodsy

Effects	**Strength**
Peaceful	○ ○ ○ ○ ○
Sleepy	○ ○ ○ ○ ○
Pain Relief	○ ○ ○ ○ ○
Hungry	○ ○ ○ ○ ○
Uplifted	○ ○ ○ ○ ○
Creative	○ ○ ○ ○ ○

Ratings ☆ ☆ ☆ ☆ ☆

Strain

Grower

Date

Acquired $

| Indica | Hybrid | Sativa |

☐ Flower   ☐ Edible   ☐ Concentrate

Symptoms Relieved

Notes

Effects	Strength
Peaceful	○ ○ ○ ○ ○
Sleepy	○ ○ ○ ○ ○
Pain Relief	○ ○ ○ ○ ○
Hungry	○ ○ ○ ○ ○
Uplifted	○ ○ ○ ○ ○
Creative	○ ○ ○ ○ ○

Ratings ☆ ☆ ☆ ☆ ☆

Strain

Grower

Date

Acquired $

| Indica | Hybrid | Sativa |

☐ Flower   ☐ Edible   ☐ Concentrate

Symptoms Relieved

Sweet
Fruity   Floral
Sour   Spicy
Earthy   Herbal
Woodsy

Notes

Effects	Strength
Peaceful	○ ○ ○ ○ ○
Sleepy	○ ○ ○ ○ ○
Pain Relief	○ ○ ○ ○ ○
Hungry	○ ○ ○ ○ ○
Uplifted	○ ○ ○ ○ ○
Creative	○ ○ ○ ○ ○

Ratings ☆ ☆ ☆ ☆ ☆

Strain

Grower

Date

Acquired

$

| Indica | Hybrid | Sativa |

☐ Flower   ☐ Edible   ☐ Concentrate

Symptoms Relieved

Notes

Sweet
Fruity
Floral
Sour
Spicy
Earthy
Herbal
Woodsy

Effects	Strength
Peaceful	○ ○ ○ ○ ○
Sleepy	○ ○ ○ ○ ○
Pain Relief	○ ○ ○ ○ ○
Hungry	○ ○ ○ ○ ○
Uplifted	○ ○ ○ ○ ○
Creative	○ ○ ○ ○ ○

Ratings ☆ ☆ ☆ ☆ ☆

Strain

Grower

Date

Acquired

$

| Indica | Hybrid | Sativa |

☐ Flower   ☐ Edible   ☐ Concentrate

Symptoms Relieved

Notes

Sweet

Fruity

Floral

Sour

Spicy

Earthy

Herbal

Woodsy

Effects	**Strength**
Peaceful	○ ○ ○ ○ ○
Sleepy	○ ○ ○ ○ ○
Pain Relief	○ ○ ○ ○ ○
Hungry	○ ○ ○ ○ ○
Uplifted	○ ○ ○ ○ ○
Creative	○ ○ ○ ○ ○

Ratings ☆ ☆ ☆ ☆ ☆

Strain

Grower

Date

Acquired

$

Indica	Hybrid	Sativa

☐ Flower   ☐ Edible   ☐ Concentrate

Symptoms Relieved

Sweet

Fruity

Floral

Sour

Spicy

Earthy

Herbal

Woodsy

Notes

Effects	**Strength**
Peaceful	○ ○ ○ ○ ○
Sleepy	○ ○ ○ ○ ○
Pain Relief	○ ○ ○ ○ ○
Hungry	○ ○ ○ ○ ○
Uplifted	○ ○ ○ ○ ○
Creative	○ ○ ○ ○ ○

Ratings ☆ ☆ ☆ ☆ ☆

Strain

Grower

Date

Acquired

$

| Indica | Hybrid | Sativa |

☐ Flower ☐ Edible ☐ Concentrate

Symptoms Relieved

Notes

Effects	Strength
Peaceful	○ ○ ○ ○ ○
Sleepy	○ ○ ○ ○ ○
Pain Relief	○ ○ ○ ○ ○
Hungry	○ ○ ○ ○ ○
Uplifted	○ ○ ○ ○ ○
Creative	○ ○ ○ ○ ○

Ratings ☆ ☆ ☆ ☆ ☆

Strain

Grower

Date

Acquired

$

| Indica | Hybrid | Sativa |

☐ Flower   ☐ Edible   ☐ Concentrate

Symptoms Relieved

Notes

Sweet
Fruity
Floral
Sour
Spicy
Earthy
Herbal
Woodsy

Effects	Strength
Peaceful	○ ○ ○ ○ ○
Sleepy	○ ○ ○ ○ ○
Pain Relief	○ ○ ○ ○ ○
Hungry	○ ○ ○ ○ ○
Uplifted	○ ○ ○ ○ ○
Creative	○ ○ ○ ○ ○

Ratings ☆ ☆ ☆ ☆ ☆

Strain

Grower

Date

Acquired

$

| Indica | Hybrid | Sativa |

☐ Flower ☐ Edible ☐ Concentrate

Symptoms Relieved

Notes

Sweet
Fruity
Floral
Sour
Spicy
Earthy
Herbal
Woodsy

Effects	Strength
Peaceful	○ ○ ○ ○ ○
Sleepy	○ ○ ○ ○ ○
Pain Relief	○ ○ ○ ○ ○
Hungry	○ ○ ○ ○ ○
Uplifted	○ ○ ○ ○ ○
Creative	○ ○ ○ ○ ○

Ratings ☆ ☆ ☆ ☆ ☆

Strain

Grower

Date

Acquired

$

| Indica | Hybrid | Sativa |

☐ Flower   ☐ Edible   ☐ Concentrate

Symptoms Relieved

Notes

Effects	**Strength**
Peaceful	○ ○ ○ ○ ○
Sleepy	○ ○ ○ ○ ○
Pain Relief	○ ○ ○ ○ ○
Hungry	○ ○ ○ ○ ○
Uplifted	○ ○ ○ ○ ○
Creative	○ ○ ○ ○ ○

Ratings ☆ ☆ ☆ ☆ ☆

Strain

Grower

Date

Acquired $

| Indica | Hybrid | Sativa |

☐ Flower   ☐ Edible   ☐ Concentrate

Symptoms Relieved

Sweet
Fruity   Floral
Sour   Spicy
Earthy   Herbal
Woodsy

Notes

Effects	Strength
Peaceful	○ ○ ○ ○ ○
Sleepy	○ ○ ○ ○ ○
Pain Relief	○ ○ ○ ○ ○
Hungry	○ ○ ○ ○ ○
Uplifted	○ ○ ○ ○ ○
Creative	○ ○ ○ ○ ○

Ratings ☆ ☆ ☆ ☆ ☆